# Manual of Infertility

61st AICOG BHUBANESWAR 2018

# Manual of Infertility

*Editors*

**SN Tripathy**
**KC Mahapatra**
**SK Giri**
**Nandita Palshetkar**
**Babita Panda**

JAYPEE *The Health Sciences Publisher*
New Delhi | London | Panama

**Jaypee Brothers Medical Publishers (P) Ltd**

**Headquarters**

Jaypee Brothers Medical Publishers (P) Ltd
4838/24, Ansari Road, Daryaganj
New Delhi 110 002, India
Phone: +91-11-43574357
Fax: +91-11-43574314
Email: jaypee@jaypeebrothers.com

**Overseas Offices**

J.P. Medical Ltd
83 Victoria Street, London
SW1H 0HW (UK)
Phone: +44-20 317 08910
Fax: +44 (0)20 3008 6180
Email: info@jpmedpub.com

Jaypee-Highlights Medical Publishers Inc
City of Knowledge, Bld. 235, 2nd floor, Clayton
Panama City, Panama
Phone: +1 507-301-0496
Fax: +1 507-301-0499
Email: cservice@jphmedical.com

Jaypee Brothers Medical Publishers (P) Ltd
17/1-B Babar Road, Block-B, Shyamoli
Mohammadpur, Dhaka-1207
Bangladesh
Mobile: +08801912003485
Email: jaypeedhaka@gmail.com

Jaypee Brothers Medical Publishers (P) Ltd
Bhotahity, Kathmandu, Nepal
Phone: +977-9741283608
Email: Kathmandu@jaypeebrothers.com

Website: www.jaypeebrothers.com
Website: www.jaypeedigital.com



**Inquiries for bulk sales may be solicited at:** jaypee@jaypeebrothers.com

***Manual of Infertility***

First Edition: **2018**

ISBN 978-93-5270-371-5

*Printed at: Samrat Offset Pvt. Ltd.*

# Contributors

**Anuradha Tibrewal**
Consultant
Raipur, India

**Babita Panda** MD
Professor and Head
Department of Infertility unit
IMS and Sum Hospital
Bhubaneswar, Odisha, India

**Kamini Rao** DGO DORCP DCh FRCOG (UK) MCh (UK) FICOG PGDMLE (Law) FNAMS
Medical Director
Milann—The Fertility Center
A Unit of BACC Healthcare Pvt Ltd
Bengaluru, Karnataka India

**Kanchana Devi**
Senior Consultant
Department of Reproductive Medicine
Cloud Nine Hospital
Chennai, Tamil Nadu, India

**Lilavati Guru**
Cuttack, Odisha, India

**Raju Nair**
Medical Director
Department of Reproductive Medicine
Mitera Hospital
Kottayam, Kerala, India

**Saubhagya Kumar Jena**
Additional Professor
All India Institute of Medical Sciences
Bhubaneswar, Odisha, India

**Siddhartha Chatterjee**

**Subhashree Rout**

**Sujata Pradhan** MD
Associate Professor
IMS and Sum Hospital
Bhubaneswar, Odisha, India

**Supriya Pani** MD
Bhubaneswar, Odisha, India

**Taswin Kaur**

# Message

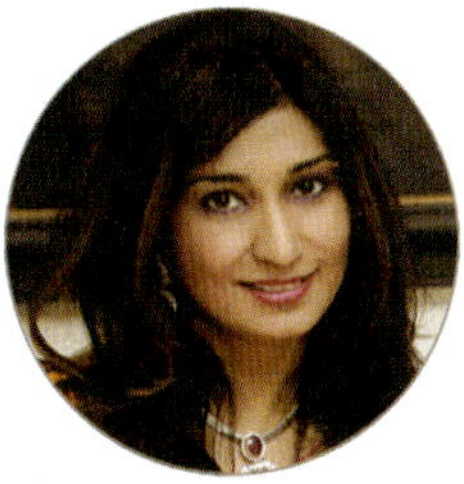

**Rishma Dhillon Pai**
MD DNB FCPS DGO FICOG
President, FOGSI—2017
Consultant Gynecologist
Jaslok Hospital, Lilavati Hospital and Hinduja Healthcare (Khar),
Bloom IVF Centre,
The Every Woman Clinic,
Mumbai, Maharashtra, India

*"Wisdom.... comes not from age, but from education and learning."*
*Anton Chekhov*

Life is a continuous process of learning. Especially in the field of medicine, which is constantly changing, it is very important to keep oneself abreast with the latest developments. It is heartening to note that academic workshop manuals are being released at the AICOG, Bhubaneswar, Odisha, India, for the benefit of the participating delegates and present varied updates in the field. Many different Manuals are being released on important subjects such as *3D Laparoscopy and Operative Oncology, Genetics, Fetal Medicine and Color Doppler, Postpartum Hemorrhage and High-Risk Pregnancy, Hysteroscopy,* etc.

I thank all the authors, for their immense contributions in building up the content for the manuals for Federation of Obstetric and Gynaecological Societies of India (FOGSI) by sharing their rich experiences in the field. These will be a big help to young gynecologists, who are still acquiring skills in various aspects of obstetrics and gynecology and a quick update for the seniors.

I extend congratulations to the organizing team of the AICOG 2018 and the editors of these manuals and wish you all success for this mega event.

*"You cannot open a book without learning something."*
*—Confucius*

# Message

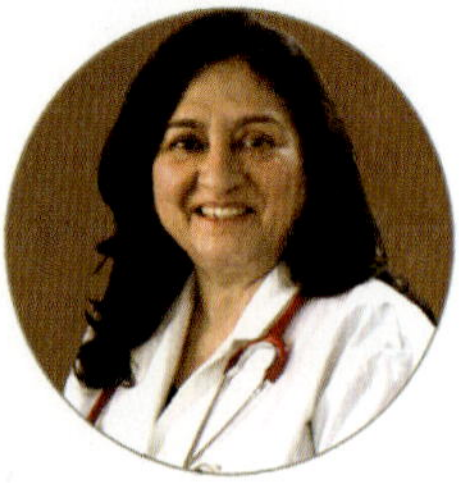

**Jaideep Malhotra**
MD FICMCH FICS FMAS FRCOG FICOG FRCPI FIAJAGO
Consultant ART (IVF)
President Elect, FOGSI—2018
Director, Rainbow IVF
Agra, Uttar Pradesh, India

*"Education is greatest gift of life, it should never stop."*

The subject of obstetrics and gynecology needs extreme proficiency as it deals with the medical specialties that focus on two different aspects. First one includes the care of pregnant women, the unborn baby, labor and delivery, as well as the immediate period following childbirth. Second aspect includes dealing with any ailment concerning the female reproductive organs. Hence, the manuals will help all those who are looking forward to gain excellence in the field of woman health. The manuals have tried to address all the issues a doctor needs.

With increasing expertise in all fields, the surgeon therefore while exercising a choice needs to follow the Hippocratic dictum—*"First, do no harm."*

We are thankful to all those who have incorporated their contribution by providing chapters from their research and collected scientific material and have shared their fruitful experiences for the delegates of the workshop.

As a part of my agenda for 2018, I as FOGSI President 2018, plan to work actively on QED (Quality, Ethics and Dignity) among our profession and also work towards HER (Health, Empowerment and Respect) towards our patients.

*"Knowledge is of no value unless you put it into practices."*

# Message

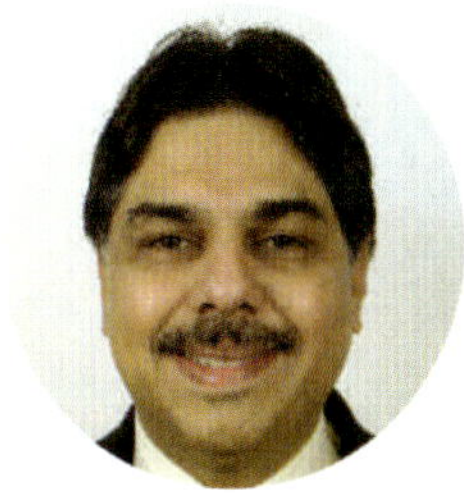

**Hrishikesh Pai**
Secretary General, FOGSI

It is my proud privilege to invite and welcome all delegates to the 61st All India Congress of Obstetrics and Gynaecology (AICOG) from 17th–21st January, 2018 at the Temple City of India, Bhubaneswar, Odisha, India.

It is propitious to note that the academic workshop manuals are being released which will reap beneficial reward to all the participating delegates.

I thank all the authors, for their immense contributions in building up the content for the manuals for Federation of Obstetric and Gynaecological Societies of India (FOGSI) by sharing their rich experiences in the field. These will be a big help to young gynecologists, who are still acquiring skills in various aspects of obstetrics and gynecology and a quick update for the seniors.

I forward my heartiest congratulations to all the contributors, the editors and the delegates of the workshop.

# Message

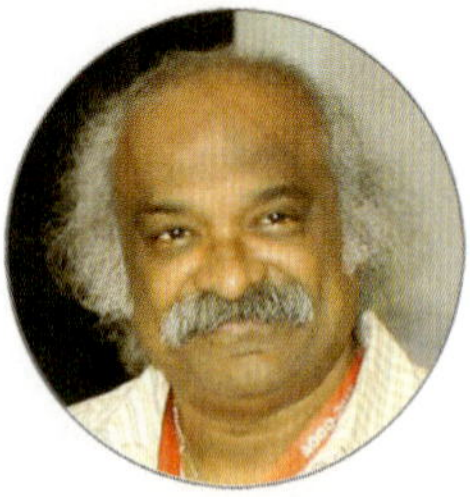

**PC Mahapatra**
Professor
Department of Obstetrics and Gynecology
SCB Medical College, Cuttack, Odisha, India
President, FOGSI—2011
Organising Chairperson

It is my proud privilege to invite and welcome all delegates to the 61st All India Congress of Obstetrics and Gynaecology (AICOG) from 17th–21st January, 2018 at the Temple City of India, Bhubaneswar, Odisha, India.

The five days of academic extravaganza will certainly enrich the scientific knowledge of all participating delegates and faculty. The precongress workshop on various aspects of this specialty will be held on 17th January 2018.

A quote by Edwin Louis Cole says that "*Winners are not those who never fail but those who never quit*" is apt for all the clinicians who are determined enough to see and overcome all the difficulties that are faced in the field of obstetrics and gynecology.

Today, with the advancement in the field of obstetrics and gynecology, everyone requires an in-depth knowledge of the complex subjects associated with the field so as to gain excellence in it.

This manual will prove to be a boon to all those who are associated with the field and wants to gain more knowledge in the subject matter.

# Message

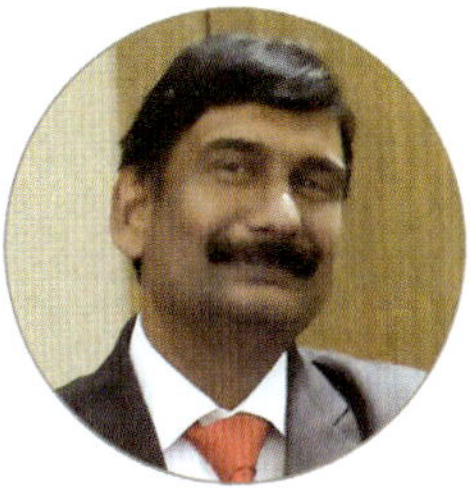

**HP Pattanaik**
Head
Department of Obstetrics and Gynecology
City Hospital
Cuttack, Odisha, India
Vice President, FOGSI—2009
Organising Secretary

Greetings from 61st AICOG 2018!
It is a matter of great pleasure to invite you all to 61st AICOG, from 17th–21st January, 2018 at the Temple City of India, Bhubaneswar, Odisha, India. The 11th Precongress workshops will be held on 17th January, 2018 in three medical colleges of Bhubaneswar.

It is propitious to note that the academic workshop manuals are being released which will reap beneficial reward to all the participating delegates.

It will also prove to be beneficial to the members of Federation of Obstetric and Gynaecological Societies of India (FOGSI), those who were unable to register themselves for the academic workshops.

I forward my heartiest congratulations to all the contributors, the editors and the delegates of the workshop.

# Preface

*'To get and beget'* is the basic human driving force. Hence infertility is a problem of immense magnitude. Infertility affects 10–15 % of couples trying to conceive. In India, one out of five couples is childless. Having a child for most individuals is an important milestone; and being unable to do so represents a major disaster.

The etiology of female infertility can be broken down into ovulation disorders, uterine abnormalities, tubal obstruction and peritoneal factors. Cervical factors are also thought to play a minor role.

The investigation of the infertile patient must begin with adequate history taking and physical examination and diagnostic evaluation of both the partners simultaneously. If the initial evaluation shows any abnormality, further investigations should be suggested according to the individual case. Proper evaluation as per guidelines helps in diagnosing cause of majority of cases. A target-oriented approach maximizes the chances of conception while minimizing the time to achieve pregnancy and treatment-related adverse effects.

At present in infertility work-up, the most neglected area is uterus, Research is necessary in the area of endometrial receptivity and on the molecular factors of the endometrium. Dilatation and curettage or endometrial aspiration should be done to exclude endometrial tuberculosis and to stimulate the good molecules of the endometrium. In 300 BC Aristotle has told, *'The womb is the field of generation; and if this field be corrupted it is invain to expect any fruit though it be ever so well sown.'*

Tubal factor accounts for 25–35% of female infertility. In addition to that a large proportion of post-sterilized females contribute to tubal factor infertility. Evaluation of the fallopian tubes is an essential part of a fertility work-up. Several non-surgical and surgical methods have been used since decades to evaluate the tubal patency. HSG has been used for a long time for assessment of tubal patency. In ultrasonography various methods like SIS, HyCoSy and HyFoSy are used for evaluation of the fallopian tube. HyFoSy allows a more accurate diagnosis of tubal patency compared with HyCoSy. Laparoscopy and dye test remains the gold standard among tubal patency tests until a suitable non-invasive test is available. In most of the infertility evaluation guidelines, tubal evaluation is the last step. The guidelines are not in agreement on the most effective diagnostic scenario for tubal evaluation.

The decision for managing a case of tubal factor infertility should be taken considering all other possible factors leading to infertility. Presently ART is widely used for treatment of tubal factor infertility, but the role of tubal reconstructive surgeries for selected cases in the hand of experts cannot be completely ignored. Tubal reconstructive surgery avoids the complications associated with ART ie. OHSS, multiple pregnancies, high risk of obstetric and perinatal complications. Surgery is less costly than ART and in the hand of experts tubal reconstruction carries a reasonable success rate for pregnancy. Surgery performed once offers the opportunity of pregnancy for multiple times.

Several treatment options have been used to overcome male infertility. Intrauterine insemination (IUI) is one of the easy, affordable and widely practiced treatment for many infertile couples. Intrauterine insemination (IUI) aims to make a reasonable fraction of motile spermatozoa available close to the oocyte around the time of ovulation. Presently global success rate for IUI has been up to 10–15%. Hence various strategies have been tried to optimize the outcome of IUI. With the advent of ICSI, severe male factor which was considered untreatable became treatable and with the parallel improvement in knowledge about genetics and advancement in molecular biology, understanding of the genetic aspect of male fertility and infertility emerged. This has opened new vistas in the assessment and treatment of male factor infertility. In any male with severe oligozoospermia or azoospermia, genetic testing must be done and it is important to continue research in this subject.

Infertility is a very sensitive social issue. The graduation in status through motherhood is so marked that barrenness is a dreaded condition. These stigmatized couples spend all their money by traveling to every nook and corner of the country where they hope to realize their dream. These childless couples use a variety of traditional, religious and herbal treatments in addition to the evidence-based medicine hoping for a miracle. There are many phages and modality of treatment for infertility, but nothing gives a good success rate, We, who are infertility specialists should take a very sympathetic attitude towards them and guide them properly, for anovulation, ovulation stimulating drugs, for tubal factor infertility, ART or tubal reconstructive surgery, for uterine factor, surrogacy or adoption and for male factor infertility IUI or ICSI.

We hope this workshop will help you a lot in infertility management.

*Blessed trinity, have pity*
*You can give the blind man sight*
*Fill the barren rocks with grass*
*Grant this house a child tonight'*

**Irish Proverb**

# Contents

# Chapter 1

# Approach to Infertile Couple: Basic Evaluation Protocol

*Sujata Pradhan*

## INTRODUCTION

Infertility is defined as inability to conceive after one year of regular and unprotected intercourse. Approximately 85% of couple conceives within one year of cohabitation. Hence infertility evaluation should start after one year. Early evaluation is required after 6 months in certain situations when female age is more than 35 years, history of oligo or amenorrhea, known uterine or tubal disease, stage III/IV endometriosis or known male subfertility.

Evaluation should start with detail history including reproductive, medical, treatment and family history of both partners. This is followed by a thorough physical examination to document any specific finding pertaining to a suggestive history.

Diagnostic evaluation of the couple should be precise, specific and cost effective with initial importance on less invasive tests. Basic evaluation includes tests for both male and female partner.

## EVALUATION OF OVULATORY DYSFUNCTION

A detail menstrual history gives maximum information regarding ovulatory dysfunction. Regular menstrual cycle is suggestive of ovulatory cycles but objective documentation of ovulation is preferred during evaluation. In contrary, irregular cycles, oligo or amenorrhea do not require any investigation to prove anovulation.

Tests of ovulation include a panel of tests like basal body temperature (BBT) measurement, urine LH, serum LH, sonographic documentation of ovulation and mid-cycle serum progesterone. Endometrial curettage and HP study for dating endometrium is presently considered obsolete and no longer recommended.

In patients with suspected ovulatory dysfunction, additional tests like serum TSH and prolactin should be advised as altered prolactin and thyroid hormone are likely to cause cycle irregularity. In patients with amenorrhea, estimation of serum FSH helps to differentiate ovarian failure from hypothalamic causes as the management differs for both.

In infertile females with history of oligoanovulation, failure to achieve pregnancy after three to six cycles of successful ovulation induction indicates for further investigations especially tubal patency tests and if that is done alternative treatment should be considered.

### Ovarian Reserve Tests

Assessment of ovarian reserve is not routinely recommended. It should be done in patients with risk factors for decreased ovarian reserve, e.g., age more than 35 years, history of ovarian surgery or exposure to chemotherapy or radiation, family history of early menopause and unexplained infertility. Tests of ovarian reserve include antral follicle count, early follicular phase serum FSH and estradiol, clomiphene citrate challenge test and serum AMH. Combined test of ovarian reserve test does not have added advantage over a single test. Decreased ovarian reserve does not necessarily suggest failure to achieve pregnancy, rather predicts suboptimal response to ovarian stimulation during assisted reproductive technology (ART).

### Uterine Factor Evaluation

Evaluation of uterus should aim to rule out congenital as well as acquired abnormalities having reproductive cosequences, e.g., polyp, intrauterine adhesions, myomas. Methods of evaluation include hysterosalpingogram (HSG), sonosalpingogram, 2D/3D USG and hysteroscopy. Hysteroscopy is considered as gold standard for uterine cavity evaluation whereas diagnostic hysterolaparoscopy is advised for complete evaluation of müllerian anomalies.

### Tubal Patency Tests

Tubal patency tests are indicated when there are known risk factors leading to tubal factor infertility or primary treatment modalities fail to achieve pregnancy. Tubal patency tests may include HSG, sonosalpingogram, hysterosalpingo contrast sonogram (Hycosy) or laparoscopic chromopertubation. HSG is considered as the standard diagnostic test for tubal patency with PPV and NPV of 38% and 94% respectively. All methods of tubal evaluation have technical limitations that should be considered while interpreting the results. Any ambiguity in initial tubal evaluation should be confirmed by a second and different test (ASRM practice guideline).

## EVALUATION OF PERITONEAL FACTORS

Peritoneal factor evaluation is indicated when there is suggestive history of peritoneal disease, e.g., endometriosis, pelvic inflammatory disease and pelvic tuberculosis or there is evidence of pelvic pathology in ultrasonography. Diagnostic laparoscopy is considered as the gold standard for peritoneal factor evaluation. Laparoscopy is also indicated in case of abnormal HSG, unexplained infertility and long duration infertility (>3 years) when there is no clear indication for ART.

### Male Factor Evaluation

Evaluation of male partner should be done simultaneously along with the female. Initial approach starts with detail reproductive history and analysis of at least one semen sample. Semen analysis should be done as per WHO 2010 semen analysis manual. If initial history or semen analysis reveals any abnormality, a thorough medical history, family history and physical examination is warranted by an urologist or specialist in male reproduction. Physical examination should include general examination followed by examination of external genitalia and secondary sexual characteristics.

### Role of Endocrine Evaluation in Males

Hormonal evaluation is indicated in case of decreased sperm concentration (<10 million/mL), sexual dysfunction or any feature suggestive of specific endocrinopathy. Serum FSH and total testosterone estimation is the first line of investigation. A high FSH beyond reference limit clearly suggest declining or failed spermatogenesis, while a normal FSH does not always rule out an abnormal semen analysis. If total testosterone is low, further evaluation is warranted with estimation of serum LH, prolactin and TSH.

### Genetic Screening in Male Infertility

The incidence of genetic and chromosomal abnormalities is much higher in infertile males as compared to fertile population. The commonly indicated tests for screening are peripheral blood karyotype, PCR for Y-chromosome microdeletion and CFTR (cystic fibrosis transmembrane regulator)-gene mutation in males with CBAVD (congenital bilateral absence of vas deference). The most common chromosomal abnormality associated with male infertility is sex chromosome aneuploidy (47XXY; Klinefelter syndrome).

## CONCLUSION

Initial infertility evaluation must include proper history taking, basic physical examination and diagnostic evaluation of both the partners simultaneously. If the initial evaluation shows any abnormality, further investigations should be suggested according to the individual case. Proper evaluation as per guidelines helps in diagnosing cause of majority of cases. A target oriented approach maximizes the chances of conception while minimizing the time to achieve pregnancy and treatment related adverse effects.

## FURTHER READING

1. Practice committee of the American Society of Reproductive Medicine, Diagnostic evaluation of infertile female: a committee opinion (2015).
2. Practice committee of the American Society of Reproductive Medicine, Diagnostic evaluation of infertile male: a committee opinion (2015).

# Chapter 2

# Methods of Tubal Evaluation in Infertility

*Saubhagya Kumar Jena, Subhashree Rout*

## INTRODUCTION

Evaluation of the Fallopian tubes is an essential part of a fertility workup, as tubal pathology is the cause of subfertility in 25–35% of subfertile couples.[1] Fallopian tubes are not just tubular portals, but are motile structures and have peristalsis. The tubo-ovarian relationship, tubal function in the form of tubal peristalsis, and fimbrial function are as important as patency of the Fallopian tubes for preservation of fertility. Thus, it is required to evaluate both tubal patency and potency.

Several investigations have been used since decades to evaluate the tubal patency. Only few of them can detect tubal potency. In most of the infertility evaluation guidelines, tubal evaluation is the last step. The guidelines are not in agreement on the most effective diagnostic scenario for tubal evaluation. There is no consensus on which test should initially be used and sequence of tests.[2-5]

## METHODS

Various nonsurgical and surgical investigative modalities have been reported to assess Fallopian tubes. An ideal test should correctly identify all women with tubal disease with minimal false-negative test results. Further, the tests should be cost-effective, well tolerated by the patient, and should not have any complications. However, such an ideal investigation is yet to be found. Therefore, various tests have been tried to assess the tubal status. While nonsurgical techniques such as hysterosalpingography (HSG) and ultrasound-based techniques like saline-infusion sonography (SIS) and hysterocontrast sonosalpingography (HyCoSy) are less invasive and associated with less serious risks than surgical technique such as laparoscopy and dye test (Chromopertubation). Though, the latter is considered the gold standard for

**Flowchart 1:** Decision making pathway for choice of tubal evaluation.

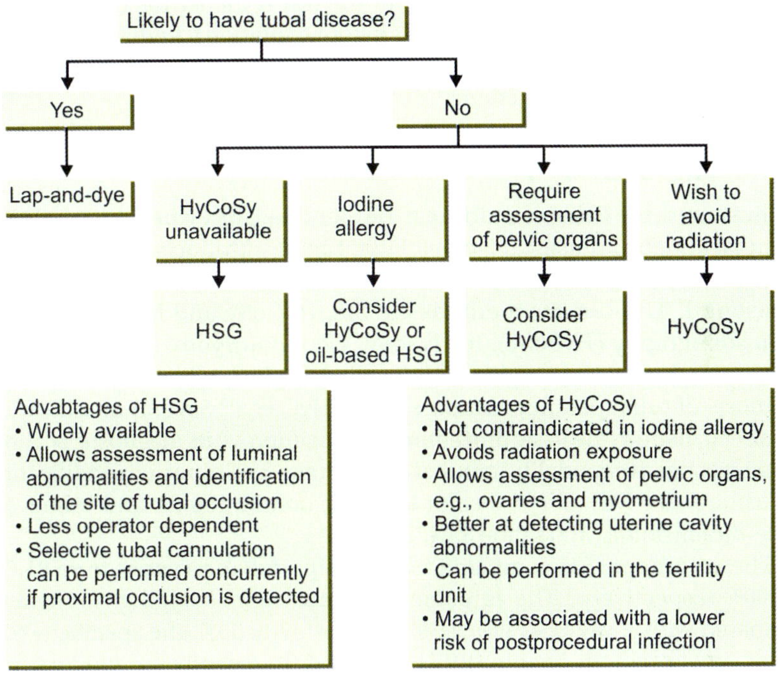


(HSG: hysterosalpingogram; HyCoSy: hysterocontrast sonosalpingography)

assessment of tubal patency and pathology. The decision making for choice of tubal evaluation is described in Flowchart 1.

## Hysterosalpingogram

It is safe, less expensive, widely available, and fairly accurate in detecting proximal tubal disease. Due to the longevity of its use, it has the largest evidence base to rule out unilateral or bilateral tubal block. The test may potentially be associated with increased pregnancy rates. Though HSG has been used for several years for tubal assessment and it has been shown in meta-analysis based on three studies gave pooled estimates of sensitivity and specificity for HSG as a test for tubal obstruction of 0.65 [95% confidence interval (CI): 0.50–0.78) and 0.83 (95% CI: 0.77–0.88), respectively. Tubal block seen on HSG will be confirmed by laparoscopy in only 38% of the women.[6] When HSG suggests that the tubes are patent, this will be confirmed at laparoscopy in 94% of the women and thus, HSG is a reliable indicator of tubal patency. These findings imply that after abnormal HSG, even in cases of bilateral pathology such as obstruction, it is still worth performing laparoscopy because, in a considerable number of these patients, the laparoscopic diagnosis allows intrauterine insemination (IUI) treatment to remain an option.[7] Due to widespread availability, it is a good screening test to rule out unilateral or bilateral tubal block. Limitations include failed catheterization or instrumentation and/or incomplete seal around the cervix, false positive due to tubal spasm or debris and reporting errors. The ideal time for the test is menstrual cycle day 7–12 (i.e. after the end of menstruation but before ovulation). Radiation exposure from this is significantly higher than that of a standard chest X-ray and there is a 1–3% risk of pelvic infection.[8]

## Sonosalpingography

In ultrasound, the Fallopian tubes can be identified only when there is fluid in the tubal lumen or outside the tubes. Fluid can be introduced using a catheter through cervix to visualize and assess the Fallopian tubes by transvaginal ultrasound. The various methods are SIS, HyCoSy and hysterosalpingo-foam sonography (HyFoSy). In HyFoSy, a nonembryotoxic gel containing hydroxyethyl cellulose and glycerol is instilled.[9] HyFoSy allows a more accurate diagnosis of tubal patency compared with HyCoSy.[10] Several modifications have been made to the basic procedure of SIS to improve its diagnostic accuracy as an investigative modality for tubal assessment. The reported modifications are using pulse Doppler and color Doppler, combining air and saline, and three-dimensional (3D) saline SSG.[1]

The accuracy of SIS compared to chromopertubation varies from 81.82% to 100% respectively.[1] The agreement of transvaginal salpingosonography compared with X-ray HSG was 94%, the sensitivity 50%, the specificity 97%, the positive predictive value (PPV) 50%, and the negative predictive value (NPV) 97%.[11] Results of SSG correlated positively with laparoscopy is 97%. SSG and HSG showed 93% correlation.[12] HyCoSy is accurate in determining tubal patency and evaluating the uterine cavity and can supplant HSG as the first-line diagnostic test in an infertility workup.[13] The shortcoming of the procedure is that even when patency of individual tube can be confirmed, it does not give any information about the site of the block, condition of the lumen, and tubo-ovarian relationship.[14]

## Laparoscopy

Currently, laparoscopy is the gold standard method. Common indications are abnormal HSG, history or symptoms suggestive of pelvic disease, previous tubal surgery, long-term infertility (>5 years), and age more than 30 years. It has certain advantages like visualization of all pelvic organs with detection and potential concurrent treatment of—(1) intramural/subserosal fibroids, (2) peritubal/periovarian adhesions, (3) endometriosis, (4) tubal constructive surgery, and (5) can be combined with salpingoscopy and/or hysteroscopy.[15-16] However, it requires general anesthesia in most cases and is associated with a 0.13% risk of bowel, urological, or vascular complications.[17]

## Salpingoscopy

Endoscopic visualization of distal tube and ampullary mucosa through distal end. It assesses internal tubal anatomy like—(1) adhesions, (2) loss of mucosal folds, (3) debris, (4) foreign bodies, and (5) abnormal vessels. Classification of salpingoscopic findings by *Brosens and Putteman*:

- *Class-I*: Normal mucosal folds
- *Class-II*: Distended fold pattern
- *Class-III*: Focal lesions like (adhesions, polyp, and strictures)
- *Class-IV*: Extensive lesions like (adhesions, polyp, and strictures)
- *Class-IVa*: With preservation of mucosal folds
- *Class-IVb*: With partial destruction of mucosa
- *Class-V*: Complete loss of pattern.

## Falloposcopy

It uses hysteroscopy to introduce flexible scope through tubal ostia to assess proximal Fallopian tube. It is therapeutic with 50% recanalization of blocked proximal tubes.

## Transvaginal Hydrolaparoscopy

This procedure involves insufflation of the pelvis with 0.4–0.6 liters of a fluid medium through an insufflating needle inserted into the posterior fornix, followed by the introduction of a small diameter rigid angled endoscope to visualize the pouch of Douglas (POD), pelvic side-walls, adnexa, and tubal patency (the dye injected transcervically). The test is performed in an outpatient setting under local anesthetic and minor operative procedures such as ovarian drilling, adhesiolysis, diathermy to endometriosis, and salpingostomy can be performed through the operative channel.[18] The single biggest risk is bowel injury, either at the time of insufflation or introduction of the endoscope. Pooled data from large case series (n = 4,232) report a rectosigmoid injury rate of 0.61%, all of which were managed either by primary repair or conservatively with no long-term sequelae.[19] The complication rate is much higher than that observed with laparoscopy and the test is not suitable for women with significant obliteration of POD due to pelvic inflammatory disease (PID), endometriosis, and fibroids.

## Fertiloscopy

It is an outpatient technique that combines hysteroscopy, transvaginal hydrolaparoscopy (TVHL), and salpingoscopy.[20] A prospective multicenter study (n = 92) reported a high degree of concordance between fertiloscopy and laparoscopy.[21] Fertiloscopy was performed first, followed by laparoscopy, by two separate operators chosen by random allocation. Videotape findings of the procedures were reviewed by two other central independent observers to resolve differences. Only 20% of women had normal findings, whereas the remainder (80%) had minor abnormalities.

### Chlamydia Antibody Test

Chlamydia trachomatis is the single largest cause of acquired tubal pathology and evidence of both current and past infection can be easily measured using *Chlamydia trachomatis* antibody test (CAT). The sensitivity (21–90%) and specificity (29–100%) vary depending on the cut-off value used to define a positive result.[22] A recent meta-analysis is evaluating the accuracy of three different CAT assays, reported a significantly better performance of MIF (microimmunofluorescence) compared to ELISA (enzyme-linked immunosorbent assay) or IF (immunofluorescence) assays.[23] The negative predictive value of the CAT is 92%, from which can be concluded that the CAT is a good test to rule out tubal pathology.[24]

## CONCLUSION

Tubal evaluation is essential in subfertile patients. Due to lack of consistency on the reported accuracy and predictive capacity of tubal patency tests, the clinical application of these tests varies widely between different centers. HSG has been used for a long time for assessment of tubal patency and is considered as the traditional standard for outpatient tubal patency testing in patients who are at low risk for tubal disease. SIS has been proved to be reliable technique for tubal evaluation. Its diagnostic accuracy can be improved using pulse Doppler and color Doppler. Introduction of ultrasound contrast media and HyCoSy have improved the visibility of the tubal lumen. HyCoSy is accurate in determining tubal patency and evaluating the uterine cavity, suggesting it could supplant HSG not only as the first-line diagnostic test in an infertility workup. HyFoSy allows a more accurate diagnosis of tubal patency compared with HyCoSy. But laparoscopy and dye test remain the gold standard among tubal patency tests until a suitable noninvasive test is available.

## REFERENCES

1. Rajesh H, Lim SL, Yu SL. Hysterosalpingo-foam sonography: patient selection and perspectives. Int J Womens Health. 2017;9:23-32.
2. ASRM Practice Committee Reports. Optimal evaluation of the infertile female. Fertil Steril. 2006;86 (5 Suppl 1):S264-7.
3. National Institute for Clinical Excellence. (2004). Fertility: assessment and treatment for people with fertility problems. [online] Available from https://www.nice.org.uk/guidance/cg11. [Accessed December, 2017].
4. Bosteels J, Van HB, Weyers S, et al. The position of diagnostic laparoscopy in current fertility practice. Hum Reprod Update. 2007;13:477-85.

5. den Hartog JE, Lardenoije CM, Severens JL, et al. Screening strategies for tubal factor subfertility. Hum Reprod. 2008;23:1840-8.
6. Panchal S, Nagori C. Imaging techniques for assessment of tubal status. J Hum Reprod Sci. 2014;7(1):2-12.
7. Watrelot A, Dreyfus JM, Andine JP. Evaluation of the performance of fertiloscopy in 160 consecutive infertile patients with no obvious pathology. Hum Reprod. 1999;14:707-11.
8. Steures P, van der Steeg JW, Hompes PG, et al. Intrauterine insemination with controlled ovarian hyperstimulation versus expectant management for couples with unexplained subfertility and an intermediate prognosis: a randomised clinical trial. Lancet. 2006;368:216-21.
9. Emanuel MH, Exalto N. Hysterosalpingo-foam sonography (HyFoSy): a new technique to visualize tubal patency. Ultrasound Obstet Gynecol. 2011;37(4):498-9.
10. Piccioni MG, Riganelli L, Filippi V, et al. Sonohysterosalpingography: Comparison of foam and saline solution. J Clin Ultrasound. 2017;45:67-71.
11. Spalding H, Martikainen H, Tekay A, et al. Transvaginal salpingosonography for assessing tubal patency in women previously treated for pelvic inflammatory disease and benign ovarian tumors. Ultrasound Obstet Gynecol. 1999;14:205-9.
12. Kore S, Hegde A, Nair S. Sonography for assessment of tubal patency: Our experience. J Obstet Gynecol India. 2000;50:63-6.
13. Lucaino DE, Exacoustos C, Johns DA. Transabdominal saline contrast sonohysterography: Can it replace hysterosalpingography in low resource countries? Am J Obstet Gynecol. 2011;204:79.
14. Seal SL, Ghosh D, Saha D. Comparative evaluation of sonosalpingography, hysterosalpingography and laparoscopy for determination of tubal patency. J Obstet Gynecol India. 2007;57:158-61.
15. Perquin DA, Dorr PJ, de Craen AJ, et al. Routine use of hysterosalpingography prior to laparoscopy in the fertility workup: a multicentre randomized controlled trial. Hum Reprod. 2006;21:1227-31.
16. Lijmer JG, Mol BW, Heisterkamp S, et al. Empirical evidence of design-related bias in studies of diagnostic tests. JAMA. 1999;282:1061-6.
17. Whiting P, Rutjes AW, Dinnes J, et al. Development and validation of methods for assessing the quality of diagnostic accuracy studies. Health Technol Assess. 2004;8:iii1-iii234.
18. Andersen AN, Goossens V, Gianaroli L, et al. Assisted reproductive technology in Europe, 2003. Results generated from European registers by ESHRE. Hum Reprod. 2007;22:1513-25.
19. Merkus JM. Fertility treatments: possibilities for fewer multiple births and lower costs–the "Umbrella" study. Ned Tijdschr Geneeskd. 2006;150:1162-4.
20. The Dutch Healthcare Authority. (2009). Diagnosis treatment combinations. [online] Available from http://ctg.bit-ic.nl/Nzatarieven/top.do. [Accessed December, 2017].
21. Jacobson TZ, Duffy JM, Barlow D, et al. Laparoscopic surgery for subfertility associated with endometriosis. Cochrane Database Syst Rev. 2010;1:CD001398.
22. Council for Public Health and Healthcare (Raad voor de Volksgezondheid en zorg). (2006). Sensible and Sustainable Care (Zinnige en duurzame zorg). [online] Available from http://rvz.net/uploads/docs/Advies_-_Zinnige_en_duurzame_zorg.pdf. [Accessed December, 2009].
23. van der Steeg JW, Steures P, Eijkemans MJ, et al. Pregnancy is predictable: a large-scale prospective external validation of the prediction of spontaneous pregnancy in subfertile couples. Hum Reprod. 2007;22:536-42.
24. Lardenoije CM, Land JA. Chlamydia antibody testing for tubal factor subfertility. Ned Tijdschr Geneeskd. 2007;151(36):1981-5.

# Chapter 3

# Evaluation of Female Infertility

*Supriya Pani*

## INTRODUCTION

Infertility is defined as the inability to achieve pregnancy after one year of regular unprotected intercourse. Evaluation may be initiated sooner in patients who have risk factors for infertility like endometriosis, polycystic ovarian syndrome (PCOS), pelvic infection or if the female partner is older than 35 years.

The primary aim of the investigation of infertility is to provide an accurate diagnosis in a manner that is rational and performed with a minimum of intervention within a limited timeframe. It is often not until a diagnosis is reached that the couple can be given an accurate diagnosis. This prognosis may have far-reaching implication for the couple including emotional and financial issues.

The etiology of female infertility can be broken down into ovulation disorders, uterine abnormalities, tubal obstruction and peritoneal factors. Cervical factors are also thought to play a minor role. The investigation of the infertile patient must begin with adequate history taking and physical examination. Evaluation of an infertile female can be done broadly under:
- Clinical evaluation
- Ovulation monitoring
- Assessment of tubal patency.

## CLINICAL EVALUATION

Clinical evaluation includes history and clinical examination:
- Age of woman is the most important determinant of fertility. Conception rates are considerably reduced by 35 years of age or more.

- Duration of marriage if more than 7 years may indicate an obstinate infertility factor.
- *Detailed menstrual history:* Delayed cycles may indicate PCOS, secondary amenorrhea responding to withdrawal treatment may be due to premature ovarian failure, and dysmenorrhea may be due to endometriosis.
- Timing and frequency of intercourse, and previous use of contraception should also be noted.
- Outcome of previous pregnancies in case of secondary infertility.

A physical examination should also be performed at the initial consultation and should include the following:

- Weight and body mass index
- Vital signs
- Thyroid palpation
- Hair distribution whether normal or abnormal
- Any signs of endocrine disease like acanthosis nigricans (a marker of insulin resistance)
- Pelvic examination to note any abnormalities of cervix and vagina, uterine size and mobility, adnexal masses or tenderness, any tenderness or nodularity in cul-de-sac.
- Pap smear can be done if not performed within previous 12 months.

## INVESTIGATIONS

Apart from routine investigations, certain special tests are to be done:

- Fasting and post-glucose should be done in PCOS cases.
- Screening for reproductive tract infections like *Chlamydia*, tuberculosis, hepatitis B and C viruses, and human immunodeficiency virus should be done.
- Endocrinological investigations, if indicated should be done.
- *Serum thyroid-stimulating hormone (TSH):* Thyroid dysfunction is common in women of reproductive age and both hyperthyroidism and hypothyroidism may interfere with reproductive function. Even a slight reduction in TSH may be associated with increased neurological problems in the offspring of these women.
- *Serum prolactin:* Hyperprolactinemia may lead to amenorrhea and anovulation. Prolactin level in serum should be measured under basal conditions and the normal range is 30–40 ng/mL. Almost all of the patients with an elevated level of prolactin have galactorrhea. Hyperprolactinemia if detected should be treated.
- *Serum follicle-stimulating hormone (FSH)* should be performed on any patient when fertility treatment is done. A day 3 FSH level is a widely accepted measure of ovarian reserve. It is particularly important in older women (older than 35 years of age), when there is history of ovarian trauma from surgery, infection or endometriosis or when there is previous poor response to fertility medications. A day 3 FSH level more than 10 mIU/mL is evidence of impaired ovarian reserve. In patients with amenorrhea, a

serum FSH level differentiates patients with ovarian failure (high FSH level) from those with hypothalamic dysfunction (low FSH level). A high serum level of FSH more than 30–40 mIU/mL with low estradiol level helps in diagnosing ovarian failure. Some patients of PCOS have elevated luteinizing hormone level in comparison with their FSH level. These patients are at risk of ovarian hyperstimulation during fertility treatment.
- *Anti-Müllerian hormone (AMH)* test is a test for ovarian reserve that should be done in women above 35 years and also in cases with low AFC. It helps in diagnosing premature ovarian failure and also in severe endometriosis with previous surgeries for ovarian cysts. It can be done at any day of menstrual cycle.
- *Serum dehydroepiandrosterone (DHEA)* is estimated in cases of PCOS. High levels of DHEA in addition to infertility causes unwanted symptoms like acne, irregular periods, head hair loss, excessive body or facial hair growth.
- *Ultrasonography (USG)*: Transvaginal sonography is the gold standard in the evaluation of female infertility. A detailed scan of the uterus and ovaries can be done. The timing of USG can be anytime during the menstrual cycle though a baseline scan on day 2–3 of cycle is ideal particularly in cases of PCOS. It helps in detecting some important uterine causes of infertility like leiomyoma, adenomyosis, and endometrial polyps. 3D scan is particularly useful in detecting uterine anomalies.

## OVULATION MONITORING

In approximately 20% of couples, the cause of infertility is ovulatory dysfunction. When menstrual cycle is either short or prolonged, it is often suggestive of disordered ovulation.

World Health Organization categorizes ovulatory disorders into three groups:
- Group I: Hypothalamic pituitary failure (10%)
- Group II: Dysfunction of hypothalamic pituitary axis PCOS (85%)
- Group III: Ovarian failure (5%).

Ovulation monitoring is done by folliculometry which is serial transvaginal USG to monitor the growth of follicle and also the endometrial thickness. Color Doppler helps in knowing the appropriate timing of administration of human chorionic gonadotropin (hCG) to trigger ovulation by noting the flow of blood around the dominant follicle. It also helps in knowing the blood flow to the endometrium. A luteal phase scan can be done to confirm ovulation, development of corpus luteum and endometrial thickness and pattern.

## TUBAL PATENCY TESTS

Tubal disease occurs in 15–20% of patients presenting with infertility. There are a number of investigations available to assess tubal patency:

- Hysterosalpingography (HSG) is the most widely used method of assessing tubal patency. It is an outpatient X-ray procedure involving instillation of water or oil-based contrast media into the uterine cavity. Apart from providing information about tubal patency, it also delineates the uterine cavity. It is done on day 7–9 of the menstrual cycle to evaluate the patency of the fallopian tubes and if there is block, the site can be known, whether proximal or distal. It helps in detecting uterine anomalies like bicornuate or septate uterus.
- *Laparoscopy and chromopertubation*: This procedure is the "gold standard" method of tubal assessment. Under laparoscopic vision, a solution of methylene blue is injected into the uterine cavity and fallopian tubes. Though an invasive procedure, it should be considered in women with risk factors for tubal obstruction like endometriosis, previous pelvic infection, ectopic pregnancy, etc. It has the advantage of detecting tubal patency along with tuboperitoneal defects. Hysteroscopy can also be done along with it to evaluate the uterine cavity. In case where tubal block has been known earlier by HSG, hysteroscopic tubal cannulation can be done. Endometrosis can be detected early and suitable treatment advised.
- Sonosalpingography is another method of tubal evaluation where saline is instilled into the uterine cavity through a Foley's catheter and tubal patency is established if the fluid is seen in the pouch of Douglas. Sonosalpingography can help in detecting endometrial polyp.
- *Hysterocontrastsonography (HyCoSy):* High resolution transvaginal ultrasound can be used in combination with echo-sensitive contrast agents to assess tubal patency. It has an additional benefit that it can be combined with a pelvic ultrasound assessment. 3D power Doppler imaging helps to capture a volume of contrast along the entire tube length and using surface rendering software, a 3D image of the tube with intraperitoneal spill can be obtained.

There is still much debate about the most appropriate investigations for female infertility. Ideally, in the best interests of the couple, an optimal process is one which provides a reliable diagnosis within a reasonable timeframe that affords a useful prediction regarding treatment options and prognosis.

## FURTHER READING


1. Crosignani PG, Rubin BL. Optimal use of infertility diagnostic tests and treatments. Hum Reprod. 2000;15(3):723-32.
2. Speroff L, Glass RH, Kase NG. Clinical Gynaecology Endocrinology and Infertility, 8th edition. Philadelphia: Lippincott Williams and Wilkins; 2010.
3. Chakravarty BN. Clinics in Reproductive Medicine and Assisted Reproductive Technology. New Delhi: CBS; 2017.

# Chapter 4

# Ovarian Hyperstimulation Syndrome and It's Management

*Anuradha Tibrewal*

## INTRODUCTION

Ovarian hyperstimulation syndrome is an uncommon but serious complication associated with assisted reproductive technology (ART). Though data about true incidence is lacking but moderate to severe OHSS occurs in approximate 1% to 5% of cycles.

Symptoms are often qualified by their severity (mild, moderate, or severe) and by the timing of onset (early and late) (Table 1).

High risk patients should be identified and preventive measures should be taken.

## MANAGEMENT

Symptomatic moderate or severe OHSS is a hypovolemic hyponatremic state. It usually involves fluid replacement to maintain intravascular perfusion and supportive care. Prophylactic anticoagulant is warranted in case of severe OHSS from the time of diagnosis through the first trimester of pregnancy. Both volume expander and paracentesis or culdocentesis for the management of OHSS in an outpatient setting (severe) are recommended.

## PREVENTIVE MEASURES

- Evidence that polycystic ovarian syndrome (PCOS), elevated AMH values, peak estradiol levels, multifollicular development and a high number of oocytes retrieved increase the risk of OHSS.
- Cutoff points are AMH values >3.4 ng/mL, AFC>24, development of ≥25follicles. Estradiol value >3500 pg/mL or ≥24 oocytes retrieved are particularly associated with an increased risk of OHSS.

**Table 1:** Classification of ovarian hyperstimulation syndrome symptoms.

| *Ovarian Hyperstimulation Syndrome stage* | *Laboratory feature* | *Clinical feature* |
|---|---|---|
| Mild | Abdominal distension/ discomfort<br>Mild nausea/vomiting<br>Mild dyspnea<br>Diarrhea<br>Enlarged ovaries | No important alterations |
| Moderate | Mild feature<br>Ultrasonographic evidence of ascites | Hemoconcentration (Hct >41%)<br>Elevated WBC (>15,000 mL) |
| Severe | Mild and moderate feature<br>Clinical evidence of ascites<br>Hydrothorax<br>Severe dyspnea<br>Oliguria/anuria<br>Intractable nausea/vomiting<br>Low blood/central venous pressure<br>Pleural effusion<br>Rapid weight gain (>1 kgin 24h)<br>Syncope<br>Severe abdominal pain<br>Venous thromboembolism | Severe hemoconcentration (Hct>55%)<br>WBC>25,000mL<br>CrCl<50 mL/min<br>Cr>1.6 mg/dL<br>$Na^+$<1235 mEq/L<br>$K^+$ >5 mEq/L<br>Elevated liver enzymes |
| Critical | Anuria/acute renal failure<br>Arrhythmia<br>Thromboembolism<br>Pericardial effusion<br>Massive hydrothorax<br>Arterial thrombosis<br>Adult respiratory distress syndrome<br>Sepsis | Worsening finding |

- Evidence supports the use of ovarian stimulation protocols using GnRH antagonists in order to reduce the risk of OHSS.
- There is insufficient evidence that clomiphene independently reduces OHSS risk.
- Aspirin reduces the incidence of OHSS.
- Metfomin decreases the risk of OHSS in PCOS patient.
- Insufficient evidence to recommend coasting for the prevention of OHSS.
- Use of a GnRH agonist to trigger oocyte maturation prior to oocyte retrieval in order to reduce the risk of OHSS.

- Live-birth rates are lower in fresh autologous cycles after GnRH trigger, but not donor-recipient cycles.
- Reproductive outcomes are improved when a low dose of HCG is coadministered at the time of GnRH agonist trigger for luteal support.
- Dopamine agonist administration starting at the time of HCG trigger for several days reduces the incidence of OHSS.
- IV calcium infusion lower OHSS risk.
- Cryopreservation prevents OHSS .

## CONCLUSION

1. Women at risk for OHSS should be identified prior to stimulation and protocol should be individualized to minimize the risk for OHSS (Antagonist cycle).
2. Use GnRH agonist as a trigger.
3. Use of cabergolin and cryopreservation of all embryos rather than transfer. This segmentation model should be followed to make OHSS free Clinic.

If preventive strategies are not effective and patient experiences severe OHSS, fluid resuscitation, supportive care, paracentesis and prophylactic anticoagulant are recommended.

The condition is self limiting and in patients who do not conceived typically resolves at the time of next menstruation period. In patients who do become pregnant, rising hCG level continue to stimulate the ovaries and symptoms may extend through the end of the first trimester.

Chapter 5

# Role of Tubal Reconstructive Surgery in the Era of ART

*Babita Panda*

## INTRODUCTION

Tubal factor accounts for 25–35% of female infertility. In addition to that a large proportion of poststerilized females contribute to tubal factor infertility and need sterilization reversal at some point of time. Presently assisted reproductive technologies (ART) is widely used for treatment of tubal factor infertility, but the role of tubal reconstructive surgeries for selected cases in the hand of experts cannot be completely ignored.

## TYPES OF TUBAL RECONSTRUCTIVE SURGERY

Tubal surgeries are planned based on the types of tubal factor abnormalities. Proximal tubal block accounts for 10–25% of tubal disease as may be due to mucus plug, debris or functional spasm causing cornual block. Other organic fibrotic lesions due pelvic inflammatory disease (PID), endometriosis and salpingitis isthimica nodosa also contribute to proximal tubal blockade. Hysteroscopic tubal cannulation is the primary surgical approach for proximal tubal block provided the distal part of the tube appears disease free. If the block is not overcome by gentle pressure, resection of the diseased portion and microsurgical anastomosis may be the next surgical option.

Distal tubal diseases may be in the form of fimbrial coagulation leading to narrow fimbrial opening or fimbrial phimosis or complete fimbrial occlusion causing hydrosalpinx. Fimbrioplasty is the procedure of choice for fimbrial coagulation in which the narrow tubal opening is dilated and the fimbria then is sutured and fixed to the tubal serosa (Bruhat procedure). Management of hydrosalpinx depends on the extent of tubal damage. Good prognosis cases with flimsy adnexal adhesion, hydrosalpinx less than 3 cm, thin and pliable tubes and preserved tubal mucosa are suitable for surgical correction.[1]

Laparoscopic neosalpingostomy is the procedure of choice for such cases as the spontaneous conception rate after surgery is as good as 58–77%.[2] In poor prognosis cases when there is dense adnexal adhesion, grossly dilated tubes with thick and rigid walls and damaged tubal mucosa reconstructive surgery does not offer significant benefit in terms of spontaneous pregnancy rate. In these cases salpingectomy followed by ART offers better prognosis.

The third category of couples with tubal factor infertility are following tubal sterilization and willing for tubal recanalization. This can be done by minilaparotomy or laparoscopy. Laparoscopic tubal recanalization needs high level of surgical expertise and is practiced by few in present day.

## WHEN TO PLAN FOR TUBAL SURGERY?

Before planning for any treatment a number of factors are taken into account, e.g. female age, ovarian reserve, presence of other contributing factors for infertility, extent of tubal damage, husband's semen analysis, and availability of surgical expertise and facility for ART. Tubal reconstruction is preferred in young age, good ovarian reserve, mild tubal damage, absence of other female infertility factors, normal semen analysis and required surgical expertize available.

## WHEN TO GO FOR ART?

Assisted reproductive technology (ART) is considered as the best treatment in advanced age, decreased ovarian reserve, extensive tubal damage, in presence of other factors contributing to infertility or abnormal male factor. Availability of appropriate facility for ART is the basic requirement before suggesting ART for any couple. When surgeons well versed with required skill for tubal reconstructive surgeries are not available ART remains the best option even when tubes are amenable for surgical repair.

### Advantages of Surgery over ART

Tubal reconstructive surgery avoids the complications associated with ART, e.g. ovarian hyperstimulation syndrome (OHSS), multiple pregnancies, high risk of obstetric and perinatal complications. Surgery is less costly than ART and in the hand of experts tubal reconstruction carries a reasonable success rate for pregnancy. Surgery performed once offers the opportunity of pregnancy for multiple times. When facility for ART is not available, surgery remains as the only option for the couple.

### Advantages of ART over Tubal Surgery

Assisted reproductive technology remains the best option in advanced age and in presence of multiple infertility factors. Surgical and anesthesia risks are avoided as well as higher risk of ectopic pregnancy. The risk of ectopic pregnancy in ART is approximately 2% versus 2–10% following tubal reconstructive surgery.[3] The higher cost of ART as compared to surgical management can be reconsidered in the present era of low cost in vitro fertilization (IVF) which offers reasonable chances for pregnancy as conventional IVF.

## CONCLUSION

The decision for managing a case of tubal factor infertility should be taken considering all other possible factors leading to infertility. The risk and benefits of both the treatment options should be considered as well. While ART is widely used for management of tubal factor, reconstructive surgery needs surgical expertise and has become a lost art. The recent trend of low cost IVF should be considered and reviewed while comparing ART and tubal surgery from financial point of view.

## REFERENCES

1. American fertility society classification of adnexal adhesions, distal tubal occlusion, tubal occlusion secondary to tubal ligations, tubal pregnancies, Mullerian anomalies and intrauterine adhesions. Fertil Steril. 1988;49:944-55.
2. Nackley AC, Muasher SJ. The significance of hydrosalpinx in in-vitro fertilization. Fertil Steril. 1998;69:373-84.
3. Practice committee of the American Society of Reproductive Medicine. The role of tubal surgery in the era of ART. Fertil Steril. 2015;103(6):e37-43.

# Chapter 6

# Role of Pre-IVF Hysteroscopy

*Raju Nair*

## INTRODUCTION

Even after lot of scientific developments and newer research into the field of reproductive medicine, the live birth is still around 30–40%. So, the scientific society is in close contest to find out methods to improve the implantation rate and improve the live birth rate (LBR). Recent developments in science proved that 60–70% if implantation failure is due to defects in the embryo development and genetic makeup of embryo. But intrauterine pathology has been reported in up to 25% of infertile women having in vitro fertilization (IVF) treatment and in as many as 50% of women with recurrent implantation failure. Even though the incidence due to uterine factor and endometrial factor is around 25%, still it is a debatable issue to find out which is the better way to identify endometrial factors of implantation failure. One of the methods advocated for the assessment of uterine cavity and endometrium is hysteroscopic assessment of uterine cavity to enhance the implantation process in an IVF cycle.

Currently, the gold standard technique for uterine factor evaluation is hysteroscopy. Hysteroscopy allows visual assessment of the cervical canal and uterine cavity and provides the opportunity to operate in the same setting; since it enables direct visualization of the uterine cavity and its relevant pathological disorders. Routine outpatient hysteroscopy before starting IVF has been postulated to diagnose and treat abnormalities of the cervix and uterine cavity and hence improve IVF outcome.

The concept of the "patient tailored approach" and the increasing interest and clinical relevance in shortening time to pregnancy clearly explain why fertility specialists has been re-evaluating the clinical relevance of hysteroscopy in the diagnosis and treatment of uterine factors and its role in the infertility workup.

The mechanism by which hysteroscopy enhance the implantation process is a debatable issue. The proposed theories are: (1) since a difficult embryo transfer procedure could compromise IVF outcome, hysteroscopy is postulated to facilitate future embryo transfer via amelioration of cervical canal obstruction and optimization of embryo transfer procedure, and thus improve treatment outcome. (2) Hysteroscopy has been proposed to improve IVF outcome by stimulation of the endometrium through surface injury, which is suggested to increase embryo implantation in the subsequent IVF treatment cycle. (3) Hysteroscopic procedure identifies the missed uterine abnormalities and a pre-IVF hysteroscopy helps in correcting the missed endometrial lesions like polyps, adhesions, etc. so that implantation happens in a better way. But in the evidence-based medicine is found difficult to substantiate these postulations.

The use of hysteroscopy as a routine procedure in the infertility workup is still under debate and there is no consensus on its efficacy and effectiveness in improving the prognosis of infertile couples. The NICE guidelines on fertility assessment and treatment state that women should not be offered hysteroscopy on its own as part of the initial investigation unless clinically indicated, because the effectiveness of this technique on improving reproductive outcome has not been established. Recently two well-designed randomized trials have published which also proves that role of pre-IVF hysteroscopy is not beneficial.

In The Lancet, two studies address the importance of the morphological evaluation of the uterus through assessment of the effect of office hysteroscopy on IVF outcomes in women undergoing IVF for the first time (inSIGHT trial) and in women with recurrent implantation failure (TROPHY trial). The authors of both studies conclude that hysteroscopy is not effective to increase the success of IVF.

In the inSIGHT trial of hysteroscopy before the first IVF cycle, Janine G Smit and colleagues randomly assigned 373 women to receive hysteroscopy 1-3 months before IVF and 377 to receive IVF without any hysteroscopy.[1] Intrauterine abnormalities were found in 37 (10%) women, as expected and most were treated for these abnormalities during the procedure. More than half of women in each group became pregnant during the trial [211 (57%) vs 203 (54%), respectively] and no differences were found between groups in ongoing pregnancies resulting in live births at 18 months follow-up [relative risk 1·06, 95% confidence interval (CI) 0·93–1·20; $p = 0{\cdot}41$].

In the TROPHY trial of women with recurrent implantation failure (after two to four IVF cycles), Tarek El-Toukhy and colleagues randomly assigned 350 women to hysteroscopy and 352 to control.[2] The investigators reported that 85 (26%) women had uterine defects, an expected proportion when cervical defects and small anatomical changes are recorded, but true intracavitary defects were seen in 34 (11%) of the women in the trial. 29% of women in each group had a live birth, with no difference between either group (relative risk 1·0; 95% CI 0·79–1·25; $p = 0{\cdot}96$).

In another systematic review, Sardo et al. on this same issue; the summary of the meta-analysis says that there is no evidence about the role of hysteroscopy as a basic infertility evaluation tool;[3] it is unclear whether hysteroscopy, performed before IVF, regardless of intrauterine abnormalities, improves LBR because of the very low-quality evidence; there is moderate quality evidence that hysteroscopy increases pregnancy rate if performed before IVF, regardless of intrauterine abnormalities; they found low-quality evidence that hysteroscopy may increase pregnancy rate when removing submucosal fibroids or endometrial polyps. No studies were found that looked at LBR when hysteroscopy was performed to remove submucosal fibroids or endometrial polyps.

These studies look only at the morphological aspects of the uterus but, functionality also needs to be explored. Recent studies using a transcriptomic analysis of the endometrium have shown that as many as 25% of women with repeated implantation failure have a displaced window of implantation.

In summary, results of these two randomized clinical trials and the meta-analysis suggest that there is no reason to perform hysteroscopy before IVF, irrespective of whether the woman is about to undergo the first cycle of IVF or if she has undergone several failed IVF attempts, if conventional transvaginal ultrasound shows no uterine pathology. Hysteroscopy does not seem to improve implantation.

## REFERENCES

1. Smit JG, Kasius JC, Eijkemans MJ, et al. Hysteroscopy before in-vitro fertilisation (inSIGHT): a multicentre, randomised controlled trial. Lancet. 2016;387(10038):2622-9.
2. El-Toukhy T, Campo R, Khalaf Y, et al. Hysteroscopy in recurrent in vitro fertilisation failure (TROPHY): a multicentre randomised controlled trial. Lancet. 2016;387(10038):2614-21.
3. Di Spiezio Sardo A, Di Carlo C, Minozzi S, et al. Efficacy of hysteroscopy in improving reproductive outcomes of infertile couples: a systematic review and meta-analysis. Hum Reprod Update. 2016;22:479-96.

# Chapter 7

# Sperm Function Tests and Its Implications

*Babita Panda*

## INTRODUCTION

Sperm function tests assess the presence or absence of factors needed for proper fertilization and initiation of embryogenesis. These tests measure the ability of a sperm to deliver a normal haploid compliment of chromosome to an ovum.[1] Practical definition of sperm function test is the test that evaluates one or more of the cellular processes exhibited by spermatozoa from the time of ejaculation to fertilization.

There are some limitations of current semen testing. A significant overlap in sperm concentration, motility, and morphology between fertile and infertile men has been demonstrated. In addition, standard measurements may not reveal subtle sperm defects such as deoxyribonucleic acid (DNA) damage but these defects can affect fertility. New markers are needed to better discriminate infertile men from fertile ones, predict pregnancy outcome in the female partner and calculate the risk of adverse reproductive events.

## FUNCTIONAL ABNORMALITIES

Three types of functional abnormalities are being currently assessed. These tests are performed when normal semen analysis reveals decreased or abnormal motility, abnormal morphology or repeated fertilization failure of intrauterine insemination (IUI) or in vitro fertilization (IVF) procedures.[2] Common specific functional tests performed are:

1. Tests for sperm viability, performed when there is poor progressive motility or higher percentage of immotile sperms
2. Test for acrosomal integrity
3. Tests for nuclear DNA fragmentation.

Apart from these tests, additional functional tests like molecular genetics testing and measurement of reactive oxygen species (ROS).[2]

## Sperm Viability Test

Absence of motility indicates that the sperms may or may not be viable. A sperm may be living, but immotile and also a sperm may be dead and immotile. These two conditions can be differentiated by hypo-osmotic swelling test (HOST).[3] In this test, the sperms are placed in hypo-osmotic solution and incubated in carbon dioxide incubator for half an hour. Influx of the fluid due to hypo-osmotic stress causes the sperm tail to coil and balloon or "swell". If more than 58% (WHO laboratory manual, 2010) are swollen, it indicates the presence of sperms having a functional and intact plasma membrane. On the other hand, if less than 58% of the sperms exhibit these changes then they are dead and immotile. HOST can be used in andrology laboratories. Such a sample after the test cannot be used for IUI, IVF or intracytoplasmic sperm injection (ICSI) (Figs. 1A to G).

## Test for Acrosomal Integrity

The physiological acrosome reaction occurs at the zona pellucida after sperm binding. Exocytosis of acrosin from the acrosomal sac occurs when the sperm head comes in contact with zona pellucida. In cases of teratozoospermia and oligospermia, some men may have otherwise normal semen parameters but spermatozoa display disordered zona pellucida-induced acrosome reaction. Others may have spermatozoa that exhibit normal zona pellucida binding but have a poor zona pellucida acrosome reaction.[4] This abnormality can be assessed either by biochemical test or by polscopic evaluation.

Biochemical tests for acrosome content can be performed by: (a) triple stain technique, (b) monoclonal antibodies to acrosomal contents, (c) *Pisum sativum* agglutinin and fluorescent stain technique, (d) radioimmunoassay, and (e) clinical acrosin assay.

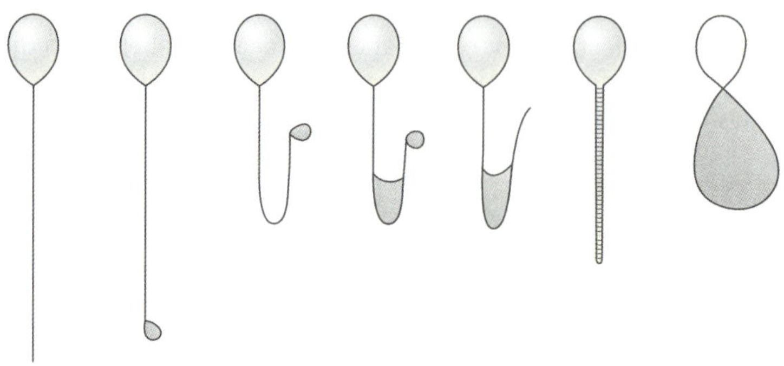

**Figs. 1A to G:** Schematic representation of typical morphological changes in human spermatozoa subjected to hypo-osmotic stress [(a): no change; (b to g): various types of tail changes. Swelling in tail is indicated by the gray area.

*Source*: Jeyendran RS, Van der Ven HH, Perez-Pelaez M, et al. Development of an assay to assess the functional integrity of the human sperm membrane and its relationship to other semen characteristics. J Reprod Fertil. 1984;70:219-28.

But, polscopic evaluation aids in identifying acrosome reacted sperms that can also be used for ICSI. The acrosome reacted sperm appears with a birefringent head. The sperm with the birefringent head can be directly used for ICSI.[5]

## Tests for Deoxyribonucleic Acid Fragmentation

Several methods have been used to test the integrity of sperm chromatin and DNA. The commonly used methods are:

- Single gel electrophoresis assay (comet assay)
- Sperm chromatin structure assay (SCSA)
- Terminal deoxynucleotidyl transferase dUTP nick end labeling (TUNEL) assay
- Halosperm test

The results of these tests are correlated with each other and with sperm morphology, motility and viability characteristics. They may provide additional information about fertilization rates with standard IVF and possibly of spontaneous pregnancy rates. The SCSA can be of predictive value for fertilization failure in vivo and in vitro.[6,7]

*Deoxyribonucleic acid fragmentation index (DFI)*: DFI indicates the cutoff value of extent of nuclear fragmentation—beyond which pregnancy even by ICSI is not possible.[8] The cutoff value has been estimated as 19%. If the level exceed 20%, the semen sample is unsuitable for fertilization.[2]

## Reactive Oxygen Species Test

In a human ejaculate, ROS are produced by both spermatozoa and leukocytes.[9,10] Seminal plasma possesses free radicals, antioxidant scavengers and antioxidant enzymes, which may be deficient in some men.[11] High ROS production may cause peroxidative damage and loss of sperm function, as well as DNA damage in both the cytoplasmic and mitochondrial genomes.[12]

Measurement of ROS:

- Direct assay
- Indirect assay.

### *Direct Assay*

- Measuring malondialdehyde (MDA) in seminal plasma is by far the most widely used direct assay as MDA is the end product of sperm of plasma membrane lipid peroxidation[13]
- Direct assay by measuring by level of 8-OH-dG which is a specific biomarker of oxidative damage to sperm DNA.[14]

### *Indirect Assay*

The most commonly used method of measurement of seminal ROS level is via indirect chemiluminescence assay. Normal ROS level in washed sperm range from 10 to 100 × $10^4$ counted photon per minute per 10 million sperm.[2]

### Microdeletion of the Y Chromosome

A wide variety of the spermatogenic defects are associated with an area of the long arm of Y chromosome (Yq11.23),[15] known as the azoospermia factor (AZF) locus. Molecular genetics testing with severe oligospermia or non-obstructive azoospermia is essential, not only because it can provide important information for the management of the patients but also because all Y-bearing spermatozoa from such men will carry the same deletion (s) and male offspring produced will be affected in the same way.[16]

## CONCLUSION

The real strength of sperm function testing lies in its ability to identify men with normal semen parameters but also who have functionally deficient spermatozoa that will fail to fertilize in routine IVF procedures. These functional deficiencies will never be observed on a routine semen analysis. As they provide a unique insight into sperm physiology, sperm function tests may also add in the designing of improved treatment protocols to be provided to the infertile couple.

## REFERENCES

1. Alukal JP, Lamb DJ. Advance tests of sperm function. Reprod Endocrinol Infertil. 2010:423-9.
2. Chakravarty BN. Clinics in Reproductive Medicine and Assisted Reproductive Technology, volume 1. New Delhi: CBS Publishsers and Distributors; 2015. pp. 36-48.
3. Avery S, Bolton VN, Mason BA. An evalution of the hypo-osmotic sperm swelling test as a predictor of fertilizing capacity in vitro. Int J Androl.1990;13:93-9.
4. Liu DY, Baker HW. High frequency of defective sperm-zona pellucida interaction in oligozoospermic infertile men. Hum Reprod. 2004;19:228-33.
5. Ghosh S, Chattopadhyay R, Bose G, et al. Selection of birefringent spermatozoa under Polscope: effect on intracytoplasmic injection outcome. Andrologia. 2012;44 Suppl 1:734-8.
6. Chohan KR, Griffin JT, Lafromboise M, et al. Comparison of chromatin assays for DNA fragmentation evaluation in human sperm. J Androl. 2006;27:53-9.
7. Evenson DP, Wixon R. Clinical aspects of sperm DNA fragmentation detection and male infertility. Theriogenology. 2006;65:979-91.
8. Fernández JL, Muriel L, Rivero MT, et al. The sperm chromatin dispersion test: a simple determination of sperm DNA fragmentation. J Androl. 2003;24:59-66.
9. Iwasaki A, Gagnon C. Formation of reactive oxygen species in spermatozoa of infertile patients. Fertil Steril. 1992;57:409-16.
10. Aitkin RJ, West KM. Analysis of the relationship between reactive oxygen species production and leucocyte infiltration in fractions of human semen separated on percoll gradients. Int J Androl. 1990;13:433-51.
11. Smith R, Vantman D, Ponce J, et al. Total antioxidant capacity of human seminal plasma. Hum Reprod. 1996;11:1655-60.
12. Sawyer DE, Mercer BG, Wiklendt AM, et al. Quantitative analysis of gene-specific DNA damage in human spermatozoa. Mutat Res. 2003;529:21-34.
13. Shang XJ, Li K, Ye ZQ, et al. Analysis of lipid peroxidative levels in seminal plasma of infertile men by high-performance liquid chromatography. Arch Androl. 2004;50:411-6.
14. Loft S, Kold-Jensen T, Hjollund NH, et al. Oxidative DNA damage in human sperm influences time to pregnancy. Hum Reprod. 2003;18:1265-72.
15. Poogothai J, Gopenath TS, Manonayaki S. Genetics of human male infertility. Singapore Med J. 2009;50:336-47.
16. Meschede D, Horst J. Genetic counselling for infertile male patients. Int J Androl. 1997;20:20-30.

# Chapter 8

# Optimizing Outcome in IUI Cycles

*Sujata Pradhan*

## INTRODUCTION

Infertility affects 10–15% of couples who have been trying to conceive. Several treatment options have been used to overcome infertility. Intrauterine insemination (IUI) is one of the easy, affordable and widely practiced treatments for many infertile couples. Intrauterine insemination aims to make a reasonable fraction of motile spermatozoa available close to the oocyte around the time of ovulation. Presently global success rate for IUI has been up to 10–15%. Hence various strategies have been tried to optimize the outcome of IUI.

Intrauterine insemination may be planned in a natural cycle or following controlled ovarian stimulation. The aim is to have at least one dominant follicle ready for ovulation. The approximate time of ovulation is estimated by various methods like ultrasonography (USG) features of the dominant follicle, urine luteinizing hormone (LH), serum LH and timing following ovulation triggering agents. Once the timing of ovulation is estimated, insemination is planned either with husband's semen sample or donor semen as in AID cycles. Semen sample is processed to isolate the total motile fraction of spermatozoa for an optimum result. The standard methods for semen preparation are density gradient and swim up method.

Outcome of IUI cycle may be affected at various steps by a number of factors contributing to the success of the cycle.

## MATERNAL AGE

Pregnancy rate after IUI cycle comes down with increasing maternal age beyond 35 years. Reported live birth rate with IUI after 40 years is 1.4–5.2%.[1]

## STIMULATION PROTOCOL

Intrauterine insemination in a stimulated cycle has better pregnancy rate than natural cycle IUI. This has been correlated to more number of dominant follicles, better endometrial thickness and correction of subtle cycle abnormalities.[2] However the difference in pregnancy rate is well marked in cases of unexplained infertility, minimal and mild endometriosis than male factor infertility. Controlled ovarian stimulation can be done with clomiphene citrate with or without gonadotropins or only with gonadotropin. Evidence shows gonadotropin stimulated cycles yield better pregnancy rate than clomiphene-induced cycles.[3] Simultaneously gonadotropins are associated with high rate of multiple pregnancy.

## NUMBER AND SIZE OF DOMINANT FOLLICLES

There has been a positive correlation between the number of dominant follicles and the pregnancy rate in IUI cycles. In a study by Kamat et al., pregnancy rate with one, two and three dominant follicles was 8.5%, 13.3% and 21.4% respectively.[4] However similar pregnancy rate has been observed when human chorionic gonadotropin (hCG) trigger was given with a dominant follicle of size 16–16.9 mm or 18–18.9 mm.[5]

## SYNCHRONIZATION BASED ON LH SURGE OR HCG TRIGGER

The Cochrane review of four randomized controlled trials (RCTs) found similar pregnancy rate when IUI was timed based on natural LH surge monitoring or following hCG trigger for oocyte maturation.[6]

### HCG Trigger versus GnRH Agonist Trigger

The same Cochrane review concluded no difference in pregnancy and live birth rate when hCG or gonadotropin-releasing hormone (GnRH) agonist is used as oocyte maturation trigger.

### Short versus Long Interval IUI

Ovulation occurs approximately 36–48 hours after HCG trigger. Hence IUI is planned mostly 36 hours after the trigger. The Cochrane review comparing short interval IUI done after 24 hours and long interval IUI done after 34–36 hours showed a higher live birth rate in later.[6] But there is no difference in pregnancy rate if insemination is done after 32–34 hours or 38–40 hours.[7]

### Single versus Double IUI

Double IUI offers better pregnancy rate than single IUI especially when done for mild male factor.[8] The NNT for one additional pregnancy was 81. Hence the extra cost, additional workload in the clinic and psychological aspect of double IUI must be considered before routine practice. In contrary pregnancy rate remains similar with single or double IUI in unexplained infertility.[9]

### Total Motile Fraction

Successful pregnancy after IUI cycle has been directly correlated to total motile fraction (TMF) of sperms. A study by Panda et al. showed significantly lower pregnancy rate when TMF was less than 5 million.[10] But maximum pregnancy rate is observed when TMF is 10–20 million and it comes down with TMF beyond 20 million due to more reactive oxygen species (ROS) produced by the spermatozoa in the prepared sample.[4]

### Luteal Phase Support

Natural cycle IUI, cycles induced with clomiphene only or clomiphene with gonadotropin do not need luteal support. However, if controlled ovarian stimulation is done with gonadotropin only pregnancy rate is higher when luteal support is given than without luteal support.[11] Different preparations of progesterone are used for this purpose.

## CONCLUSION

Young age, use of gonadotropins, more number of dominant follicles, total motile fraction more than 5 million, long interval insemination, double insemination in selected cases and use of luteal support are associated with successful IUI cycles. However, size of dominant follicles and types of trigger do not affect the outcome of IUI.

## REFERENCES

1. Nuojua-Huttunen S, Tomas C, Bloigu R, et al. Intrauterine insemination treatment in subfertility: an analysis of factors affecting outcome. J Hum Reprod Sci. 1999;180:1522-34.
2. Guzick DS, Carson SA, Coutifaris C, et al. Efficacy of superovulation and intra uterine insemination in the treatment of infertility. N Engl J Med. 1999;340:177-83.
3. Peeraer K, Debrock S, De Loecker P, et al. Low dose human menopausal gonadotropin versus clomiphene citrate in subfertile couples treated with intra uterine insemination: a randomized controlled trial. Hum Reprod. 2015;30(5):1079-88.
4. Kamath SM, Bhave P, Aleyamma TK, et al. Predictive factors for pregnancy after intrauterine insemination:A prospective study of factors affecting the outcome. J Hum Reprod Sci. 2010; 3(3): 129-34.
5. da Silva AL, Arbo E, Fanchin R. Early versus late HCG administration to trigger ovulation in mild stimulated IUI cycles: a randomised clinical trial. Eur J Obstet Gynecol Reprod Biol. 2012;164(2):156-60..
6. Cantineau AE, Janssen MJ, Cohlen BJ. Synchronised approach for intrauterine insemination in subfertile couples. Cochrane Database Syst Rev. 2014;(12):CD006942..
7. Claman P, Wilkie V, Collins D. Timing intrauterine insemination either 33 or 39 hours after administration of human chorionic gonadotropin yields the same pregnancy rates as after superovulation therapy. Fertil Steril. 2004;82:13-6.
8. Cantineau AE, Heineman MJ, Cohlen BJ. Single versus double intrauterine insemination. Cochrane Database Syst Rev. 2008;(1):CD003854.
9. Polyzos NP, Tzioras S, Mauri D, et al. Double versus single intrauterine insemination for unexplained infertility: a meta-analysis of randomized trials. Fertil Steril. 2010;94(4):1261-6.
10. Panda B, Mohapatra L, Sahu MC, et al. Success in pregnancy through intrauterine insemination at first cycle in 300 infertile couples: an analysis. J Obstet Gynaecol India. 2014; 64(2): 134-42.
11. Green KA, Zolton JR, Schermerhorn SM, et al. Progesterone luteal support after ovulation induction and intrauterine insemination: an updated systematic review and meta-analysis. Fertil Steril. 2017;107(4):924-933.e5.

# Chapter 9

# Genetic Testing of Male Factor Infertility

*Kanchana Devi*

## INTRODUCTION

With the advent of intracytoplasmic sperm injection (ICSI), severe male factor which was considered untreatable became treatable and with the parallel improvement in knowledge about genetics and advancement in molecular biology, understanding of the genetic aspect of male fertility and infertility emerged. This has opened new vistas in the assessment and treatment of male factor infertility.

Formation of a zygote and a subsequent embryo need male and female gametes. For ages the focus was on female gamete and the female partner only and since recent times the importance of male age and the sperm integrity in contributing to embryo quality has been realized.

The genetic assessment of a male is important in view of two factors: (1) Understanding the cause of poor sperm parameters and also in case of planned surgical sperm retrieval as in nonobstructive azoospermia, the probability of success of sperm retrieval through testicular sperm aspiration (TESA) can be assessed. (2) The couple gets a chance to be counseled about the chances of a child inheriting the genetic abnormality of the parent.

## GENETICS OF MALE SEXUAL DEVELOPMENT

Any embryo is bipotential in sexual development up to 6 weeks of embryonic age and after that the presence of normal Y chromosome leads to the development of male external genitalia and suppression of the müllerian duct which leads to the development of female genital tract.

## GENETICS OF TESTICULAR DIFFERENTIATION AND ITS DESCENT

In males, though the gonad (testes) initially forms in the abdominal cavity, it follows definite time line in its descent in to the scrotum.

Presence and activation of the SRY region of the Y chromosome is essential for differentiation of the gonad into male. This helps in the differentiation of primordial germ cells that migrate from the yolk sac to genital ridge to gonocytes. This along with the presence of other genes like WT1, SOX9, FGF9, and SF leads to formation of primary testicular cords with the differentiation of coelomic epithelium into sertoli cells around the gonocytes.

These genetic factors and the other factors like the gubernaculum testes, hormone testosterone, anti-müllerian hormone (AMH), and insulin-like peptide 3 (INSL3) help in the descent of the testis into the scrotum. Failure of this process leads to cryptorchidism and further loss of testicular function. Hence, the current knowledge suggests the fact that genetic factors are essential for not only sex differentiation but also the descent of the testis, which questions the practice of surgical fixing of the undescended testis for fertility purposes.

## Y CHROMOSOMAL DEFECTS AND SPERM ABNORMALITIES

The presence of SRY region in the long arm of Y chromosome which has azoospermia factor (AZF) region which in turn has three distinct regions called AZFa, AZFb, and AZFc region which code for spermatogenesis and maturation of sperms.

Micro deletion of this region leads to changes in sperm production which can vary from oligozoospermia to complete azoospermia to maturation arrest. Absence of a and b regions are associated with a poor chance to retrieve sperms from the testis. Whereas, the association of AZFc deletion, which is the commonest among the Y deletions, has a good chance of sperm retrieval by surgical techniques. Hence, assessing the genetic aspects in male factor infertility throws light on who to subject for sperm retrieval and who should be counseled for donor sperms.

*TSPY* gene in short arm of Y has been associated with initiation of meiosis in sperms.

## X CHROMOSOME DEFECTS

*AR* gene coding for androgen receptor can mutate or undergo polymorphisms resulting in androgen insensitivity. *KAL1* gene mutation of X chromosome, results in X-linked Kallmann syndrome, which manifests as hypogonadotropic hypogonadism along with anosmia. There are other genes in X chromosome like the USP26 and TAF7 gene which play a role in spermatogenesis.

### 46,XX Males

A very rare condition where the presence of SRY in the X chromosome leads to male phenotype but there is no sperm production in these men.

### Autosomal Defects

*Klinefelter Syndrome*

Klinefelter syndrome or 47,XXY karyotype is seen in 15% of men with severe sperm abnormalities. While the phenotype of a person suggests a probable diagnosis, it is important to genotype these patients as it is associated with the future risk of testicular malignancies and rapidity of sperm disappearance suggesting the possibility of sperm cryopreservation in adolescents who present early. Men who are mosaic (46,XY/47,XXY) have 25% chance of sperm retrieval and fathering a child through ICSI.

## *CFTR* GENE MUTATION

In men with congenital bilateral absence of vas deferens (CBAVD), *CFTR* gene is mutated in 60–90%. Though ICSI is an effective way to achieve fertility, transfer of mutation to offspring is a possibility. As the gene mutation not only causes infertility and is associated with other pulmonary and renal abnormalities, it is essential to screen both the partners prior to opting for ICSI.

## OTHER AUTOSOMAL GENES

*SHBG* gene, *ESR1* and *2* gene, (TA)n polymorphism, follicle-stimulating hormone (FSH) receptor gene deletion or polymorphism, autosomal homologue of *DAZ* gene called *DAZL, MTHFR* gene have all been associated with different aspects of spermatogenesis and are under evaluation for their possible roles in male infertility.

*Robertsonian translocations* occurs in 0.9% of infertile men and can be associated with a wide range of sperm picture from normozoospermia to complete absence of sperms. Risk of transmitting the translocation to offspring exists warranting the use of fluorescent in situ hybridization (FISH) technique with additional probes to rule out other translocations.

Apart from the structural and numerical defects of chromosomes, other changes like the epigenetic changes, where the deoxyribonucleic acid (DNA) sequence is retained but there is gene expression alteration, alteration in histone packing, centrosome abnormalities, and imprinting disorders are also known to affect the sperm function.

In any male with severe oligozoospermia or azoospermia, genetic testing becomes important for the above said reasons as it guides us in prognostication and in assessing the risk of transfer of these abnormalities to the offspring. It is also important to continue research in the genetics of male infertility with specific focus on impact of ethnicity on gene alterations and its consequences.

# Chapter 10

# Social and Cultural Consequences of Being Childless

*Taswin Kaur, Kamini Rao*

A wise man once said "it is hard to wait around for something that might never be; but it is harder to let go when it is everything you ever wanted".

A child—is most married couples dream; rather a family bridge. Children are usually the source of meaning in life, the ropes to strengthen the marriage bond, probably serve as insurance in old age, may be means to acquire a better life, more wealth, build useful alliances, the smile to our sorrows, and the laughter to our tears.

Being childless is a huge blow with endless consequences pictured. Infertility is a disease of the 21st century affecting more than 50 million couples worldwide.[1] In India, one out of five couples is childless.[2] Having a child for most individuals is an important life plan or rather milestone; and being unable to do so represents a major life disaster!

In a developing country like ours, both the urban and rural married women are dependent on their husbands—financially, emotionally, socially, and even spiritually. The society regards having children as the most important asset in a successful marriage. In this male-chauvinistic environment of the surroundings, women are blamed and ridiculed while men refuse to accept that they could be the root cause of being childless. In general, the society believes that men cannot be infertile so far as he can sustain an erection.[3,4] Fertility and potency are thought to be synonymous. Women fear abandonment and infidelity.[5] The woman is often judged for infertility while the men hesitate to even get tested.

In the cultural rich upbringing of ours, the existence of a joint family has taken an upper hand. The ray of the "in-law" effect further darkens the lives of these women. More often than not, these infertile women face insults, harassment, and abuse by her partner or in-laws.[6] Constant family wars are sighted as a result of the infertility blame game. Most of the women suffer from domestic violence—physical and psychological.[7,8]

In the community where childlessness is regarded as a personal tragedy, especially when related to failure to conceive or death of a child; these issueless couples tend to become socially recluse.[9] The fear or being questioned and mocked for not expanding the family makes these couples—women more often than infertile men: sorrow, frustrated, and hostile with a low self-esteem.[10-12] A study of infertile women in Ghana revealed that more than 60% of these women suffered from depression.[13] The fear of never becoming a parent makes handfuls turn to the suicidal mode.

In a female feticide rampant country, and with the typical notion of the country-men; in many instances, the absence of a male child is considered childlessness. A male child is considered as a succession of the family tree and the heir and also for ritual obligations. Jindal and Gupta's study revealed that when a couple's previous offspring was female, social pressure was the same as in cases of primary infertility.[14] The prime importance in the society for a son; as lineage, kinship, dowry, and old age concerns; makes the situation bitterer.

When viewed from the eyes of the policy makers from the national aspect; childlessness (especially, voluntary childlessness) may lead to a demographic shift where the number of old age population will outnumber the young. The decreased birth rate will lead to a negative population growth and a diminished labor force for tomorrow. However in an overpopulated country like India; this may not be of much significance.

The failure to reproduce has been negatively associated with sexual satisfaction.[15] According to studies, the prevalence of sexual dysfunction was higher in the infertile population.[16] At the end of the day, for the "barren" couple; sexual intercourse becomes mechanical and unfulfilling.[17]

In most cultures and old age customs, the inability to carry on the family line has been regarded as a serious failure on the part of the woman to fulfill her rights as a woman. Infertility often threatens the status of women in the community. Barrenness is held as a curse. Besides being inauspicious for auspicious occasions, these women are not allowed to participate in family gatherings. These women are often out casted and not recognized in their society. Studies from communities in various countries showed that these women were usually excluded from social gatherings.[18,19] In some tribes, childless men have lesser status in the society compared to their fertile peers and they are not allowed to contribute in community discussions.

The barren womb and woman is regarded as an "evil-eye".[20] These childless couples are associated with witchcraft and illnesses.

These stigmatized couples borrow and spend all the pennies they have travelling to every nook and corner where they see hope for their dream of becoming a parent may materialize.[21] Many resort to supernatural healing powers that God someday answers their dreams of having a child. These childless couples use a variety of traditional, religious, and herbal treatments in addition to the evidence-based medicine hoping for a miracle. The current cost of infertility investigations and treatment is steep. Traditional healers are more expensive than faith-based healers, but Nigerian women spend between 55% and 100% of their earnings on attempts to treat their infertility.[22] Women view childbearing as invaluable, so they are willing to prioritize treatment.

Childlessness has major social and psychological implications for the affected persons, especially in a country like India where fertility is highly valued and having children is considered urgency postmarriage. The graduation in status through motherhood is so marked that barrenness is a dreaded condition. Hence, many choose to adopt a child well before they come into the limelight for not having one. A minority of these couples accept not being a parent, as their fate and are comfortable being biologically infertile. However, for most couples—the men think of remarrying for an offspring while the women cry to sleep with the hope of having a child.

In this modern age, unknowingly motherhood is not been given utmost priority. Many women are delaying childbearing while they gain financial stability, pursue their dreams, acquire knowledge, and seek and appropriate partner.[23] Little do these women realize that their biological clock is ticking and their basket of reserved eggs are diminishing. Fertility declines with age. This increases the number of women unintentionally being permanently childless.[24]

While most couples pray and dream of a baby's cry at home; trickles of couples voluntarily choose not to become parents due to personal reasons. They are happy being childless; enjoying each other's company.[25] These cohorts of couples are said to live for the moment and have less zeal to accumulate wealth as there is no heir for their legacy. The social acceptance of these couples in this 21st century may be the green light of the disappearance of the stigmatization of being childless.

Today, assisted reproductive technology has reduced childlessness to a major extent but their success depends on an ocean of factors. Involuntary childlessness after all maximum possible efforts brings us back to the ground that in the end; we cannot play God. The reality of childlessness is complex. We as healthcare professionals, should be a shoulder for these infertile couples especially the women; reminding them that infertility is not the end of the tunnel and infertility is hope!

## REFERENCES


1. Maternal Health Task Force. (2017). The Burden of Infertility: Global Prevalence and Women's Voices from Around the World. [online] Available from: http://www.mhtf.org/2017/01/18/the-burden-of-infertility-global-prevalence-and-womens-voices-from-around-the-world. [Accessed December 2017].
2. Indiatoday. (2017). Infertility on the Rise. [online] Available from: http://indiatoday.intoday.in/story/infertility-on-the-rise/1/103037.html. [Accessed December 2017].
3. Inhorn M. "The Worms Are Weak". Men and Masculinities. 2003;5(3):236-56.
4. Mumtaz Z, Shahid U, Levay A. Understanding the impact of gendered roles on the experiences of infertility amongst men and women in Punjab. Reprod Health. 2013;10(1):3.
5. Van Balen F, Bos HMW. The social and cultural consequences of being childless in poor-resource areas. Facts, Views Vis Obgyn. 2009;1(2):106-21.
6. Wiersema NJ, Drukker AJ, Dung M, et al. Consequences of infertility in developing countries: results of a questionnaire and interview survey in the South of Vietnam. J Trans Med. 2006;4(1):54.
7. Ardabily HE, Moghadam Z, Salsali M, et al. Prevalence and risk factors for domestic violence against infertile women in an Iranian setting. Int J Gynecol Obstet. 2010;112(1):15-7.
8. Ameh N, Kene TS, Onuh SO, et al. Burden of domestic violence amongst infertile women attending infertility clinics in Nigeria. Niger J Med. 2008;16(4).375-7.

9. Papreen N, Sharma A, Sabin K, et al. Living with infertility: Experiences among urban slum populations in Bangladesh. Reprod Health Matters. 2000;8(15):33-44.
10. Doss K. Level of Depression among Infertile Women. International Journal of Psychiatric Nursing. 2015;1(1):155-6.
11. Graham M. Is Being Childless Detrimental to a Woman's Health and Well-Being Across Her Life Course?. Women's Health Issues. 2015;25(2):176-84.
12. Lakatos E, Szigeti J, Ujma P, et al. Anxiety and depression among infertile women: a cross-sectional survey from Hungary. BMC Womens Health. 2017;17(1):48.
13. Alhassan A, Ziblim A, Muntaka S. A survey on depression among infertile women in Ghana. BMC Womens Health. 2014;14(1):42.
14. Jindal UN, Gupta AN. Social problems of infertile women in India. Int J Fertil. 1989;34:30-3.
15. Wirtberg I, Moller A, Hogstrom L, et al. Life 20 years after unsuccessful infertility treatment. Human Reproduction. 2006;22(2):598-604.
16. Gremigni P, Casu G, Mantoani Zaia V, et al. Sexual satisfaction among involuntarily childless women: A cross-cultural study in Italy and Brazil. Women Health. 2016;58(1):1-15.
17. Samadaee Gelehkolaee K, Mccarthy B, Khalilian A, et al. Factors Associated With Marital Satisfaction in Infertile Couple: A Comprehensive Literature Review. Glob J Health Sci. 2015;8(5):96-109.
18. Hasanpoor-Azghdy SB, Simbar M, Vedadhir A. The Social Consequences of Infertility among Iranian Women: A Qualitative Study. Int J Fertil Steril. 2015;8(4):409-20 ,
19. Rouchou B. Consequences of infertility in developing countries. Perspect Public Health. 2013;133(3):174-9.
20. Qiu R-Z. Sociocultural dimensions of infertility and assisted reproduction in the Far East. In: E Vayena, PJ Rowe, PD Griffin (Eds). Current Practices and Controversies in Assisted Reproduction. Geneva: WHO; 2002. p. 396.
21. Widge A. Sociocultural attitudes towards infertility and assisted reproduction in India. In E Vayena, PJ Rowe, PD Griffin (Eds). Current Practices and Controversies in Assisted Reproduction. Geneva: WHO; 2002. pp.60-74.
22. Nieuwenhuis SL, Odukogbe AT, Theobald S, et al. The impact of infertility on infertile men and women in Ibadan, Oyo State, Nigeria: A qualitative study. Afr J Reprod Health. 2009;13(3):85-98.
23. Koert E, Daniluk J. When time runs out: reconciling permanent childlessness after delayed childbearing. J Reprod Inf Psychol. 2017;35(4):342-52.
24. Simoni M, Mu L, Collins S. Women's career priority is associated with attitudes towards family planning and ethical acceptance of reproductive technologies. Human Reproduction. 2017;32(10):2069-75.
25. Peterson H, Engwall K. Missing Out on the Parenthood Bonus? Voluntarily Childless in a "Child-friendly" Society. J Fam Eco Issues. 2015;37(4):540-52.

# Chapter 11

# Stress in Infertility

*Siddhartha Chatterjee*

## INTRODUCTION

It is well accepted that many body functions of an individual are controlled by that person's mind, which is called body and mind relationship. Thus, a psychological stress or unrest influences an individual's reproductive process. An individual's lifestyle is strongly associated with stress factors. Lifestyle affects fertility to a great extent. Smoking, consuming alcohol, the use of recreational drugs, so also unbalanced diet, over- or undernutrition, all influence fertility. The former three affect sperm and egg qualities, as well as the reproductive process (due to presence of cadmium and cotinine). Both underweight and overweight women suffer from hormonal dysfunctions, hypertension, recurrent spontaneous abortions (RSAs), polycystic ovarian syndrome (PCOS) and diabetes mellitus (DM). Lynch et al. in their study had shown that even preconception stress increases the risk of infertility.[1]

Infertility per se can cause psychological upset. It has been observed that 40% of infertile women meet the criteria of psychiatric disorders, as compared to 3% in community samples. Infertility along with the stress of treatment procedure can cause disturbed relationship with partners, family and friends. Infertility can raise anger in couples against close relatives, medical professional and even against God. There may be disturbed sex life due to loss of interest. The expenditure for treatment can lead to severe financial insecurities as well as poor performance in job.

Mental stress itself is an important factor for lowering the success rate in infertility treatment. More ovulatory dysfunction, tubal dysfunction, impaired spontaneity about the attempt of pregnancy can happen due to stress. Some research indicates that stress may have an impact on other aspect of infertility beyond ovulation, including problem with fertilization and implantation. Stressed individuals have less sexual arousal, and ultimately end up in treatment dropout. It has been suggested that psychological stress exerts its effect through a reduction of pulsation frequency in gonadotropin-releasing hormone (GnRH) release[2] due to increase in the level of stress hormones such as adrenaline, catecholamine and cortisol. Stress can impair not only spontaneous reproduction procedures but also the reproductive technologies. A study from the University of California, San Diego documented that in in vitro fertilization (IVF) program, less number of oocytes are obtained from women under stress. They also produce diminished number of fertilized eggs along with diminished pregnancy rates, live birth rates as well as low birth weights.[3] A study by researchers at the National Institutes of Health (NIH) and University of Oxford supports widespread belief that stress can reduce a woman's chance of becoming pregnant. The study is first of its kind to document among women without history of fertility problems and association between high level of substance indicative of stress (alpha-amylase secreted in saliva) and a reduced change of being pregnant.[4]

Another study from Israeli researchers found that when women undergoing IVF distressed by entertaining themselves by a clown, the success rate increases. In contrary to the above fact, one study has suggested that stress does not affect IVF outcome.[5]

Not only females, bur stress can affect the male factor of infertility as well. Researchers have shown that sperm count, motility and morphology can be influenced negatively by stress. It is also observed that high cortisol level due to stress can affect the process; thereby testosterone (ST) level can go down. Moreover, overproduction of oxygen free radicals leading to oxidative stress can affect sperm quality directly. A new study from University of Pennsylvania School of Medicine conducted on mice found that stress can cause permanent damage to a man's sperm and can stunt child's brain development. Enough scientific evidences exist to suggest that psychological stress can affect spermatogenesis due to varying ST secretion and due to direct inhibitory action of hypothalamic-pituitary-gonadal (HPG) axis and Leydig cells in the testes.[6]

Polycystic ovarian syndrome with infertility requires special mention, so far as stress is concerned. One of the main factors for development of PCOS is stress, though obesity and abnormal lifestyle are also responsible. The stress of studies, expectation of parents and single-child family can lead to adolescent PCOS frequently. Apart from this, adult PCOS may develop from other factors like personal relationship with kins, ill-developed mental and physical relation between the couples, poor performances in studies as well as jobs, unpleasant workplace and disharmony between colleagues. This may be frequent features in women working in information technology (IT) sectors and according to our experience, these women are the worst sufferers of stress, leading to poor sexual performance and infertility.

Another source of stress in infertility is the treatment procedure. It is observed that infertile women are scared of any interference, even from a vaginal examination or from transvaginal ultrasonography (TV-USG). Invasive procedures like laparoscopy or ovum pick-up (OPU) sometimes are unacceptable to them. Injectable like gonadotropin is another source of stress. One thing is very important that attending the fertility clinic frequently, as it is necessary for ovulation monitoring, intrauterine insemination (IUI) or IVF procedures can lead to production of stress in infertile women. When the husbands have to accompany the female partners, it causes lot of nonacceptance in male partners, as they have to face loss of job hours and long waiting in the clinics.

As medical personnel are attending the infertile population, an extensive search has been undertaken by medical personnel to find the way outs to allay apprehension of infertile couples. Primarily, psychological support in organized forms is found to be offered to the population suffering from infertility is found to be useful. Counseling is to be offered to individuals or in groups. The induction of positive approach, relaxation exercises, weight reduction, combined approach to family making are to be discussed. The development of couple communication, use of humor to reduce stress and goal setting are also important steps.[7] The couples should be taught to shake off their stress at the end of the day and do not feel worried or anxious all the time.

Psychological support in the infertility clinic is offered in an informal way. Easy and relaxed environment in the clinic along with friendly behavior from all the clinic staffs are encouraging. Help is given in decision-making. All the information is made available through website as well as discussion, and answers are provided to all questions. All telephone calls are attended with care and if necessary, counseling over the telephone is also offered. There should always be approach of tender loving care. A study has shown that decrease in stress level can lead to increase in conception rate by 34%.[8] Many are of the opinion that acupuncture and body massage may help in reducing stress. A study conducted in Germany indicated that many women underwent acupuncture treatment just before and after embryo transfer (ET) resulted in significantly higher pregnancy rate (42.5%) in treatment group, in comparison to 26.3% pregnancy rate in control group.[9]

One should offer counseling with the following ideas in mind and try to site many examples. Infertility is not a disease and it requires more supportive treatment. One should follow relaxed approach and try to be more of a friend and a guide than a doctor or a nurse. One should try to create confidence of the affected couple on the treating team as well as on themselves (self-confidence) and allay apprehensions about the treatment procedures.

One should convey to the infertile couple that pregnancy is a natural process, and the aim of the treatment should be to create an environment conducive for pregnancy to occur. One should not be crazy about pregnancy and let it happen itself naturally. Discussing personal experiences and informing case histories of the successful couples in the form of storytelling also helps to build the confidence.

Induction of positive approach is another way of psychological supportive approach. Getting up early in the morning and doing some light exercises helps a lot. Avoidance of watching television serials showing family complications, rather seeing light entertainment shows or animal world cheers up the mind. The couples should avoid discussing treatment details with everyone, and avoid involving senior members of the family in decision-making. The couples should start preparing themselves to become true parents.

## REFERENCES


1. Lynch CD, Sundaram R, Maisog JM, et al. Preconception stress increases the risk of infertility: results from a couple-based prospective cohort study—the LIFE study. Hum Reprod. 2014;29(5):1067-75.
2. Pirkalani K, Talaeerad Z, Mohammadi K, et al. Psychological stress causes relative infertility through direct change in the frequency pattern of GnRH release from the hypothalamus. Opening Lectures. 9th Congress of the European Society of Gynecology Book of Abstracts. Copenhagen, Denmark, 8-11 September, 2011. p. 241.
3. Klonoff-Cohen H, Chu E, Natarajan L, et al. A prospective study of stress among women undergoing in vitro fertilization or gamete intrafallopian transfer. Fertil Steril. 2001;76(4):675-87.
4. National Institutes of Health. (2010). NIH study indicates stress may delay women getting pregnant. [online] Available from https://www.nih.gov/news-events/news-releases/nih-study-indicates-stress-may-delay-women-getting-pregnant. [Accessed December, 2017].
5. Boivin J, Griffiths E, Venetis CA. Emotional distress in infertile women and failure of assisted reproductive technologies: meta-analysis of prospective psychosocial studies. BMJ. 2011;342:d223.
6. Nargund VH. Effects of psychological stress on male fertility. Nat Rev Urol. 2015;12(7):373-82.
7. Chatterjee S. Infertility and environment. JKIMSU. 2012;1(1):24-9.
8. Domar AD. Stress and infertility in women: is there a relationship? In Session: Psychotherapy in Practice. 1996;2(2):17-27. [online] Available from http://onlinelibrary.wiley.com/doi/10.1002/(SICI)1520-6572(199622)2:2%3C17::AID-SESS3%3E3.0.CO;2-5/full. [Accessed December, 2017].
9. Paulus WE, Zhang M, Strehler E, et al. Influence of acupuncture on the pregnancy rate in patients who undergo assisted reproduction therapy. Fertil Steril. 2002;77(4):721-4.